STAY STRONG

Kidney Dialysis
Peritoneal Dialysis
LOGBOOK

By Eloisa Bustos

Published by: Eloisa Bustos
ISBN: 978-1-387-78178-2

msha.ke/nightoferispublishing

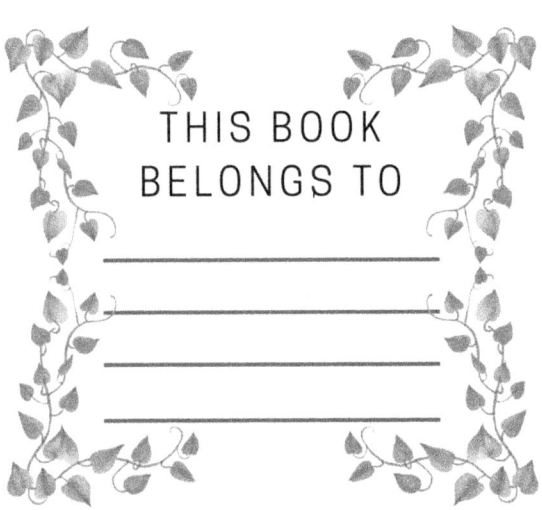

THIS BOOK
BELONGS TO

_____

_____

_____

_____

Example Page

PD Dialysis Solution Inventory

Count Start Date: __7/19/2022__ Fact #: __123456789__

Boxes															
X	X	X	X	X	X	X	X								

Solution Color: __Green__

Strength: __2.5%__

Liters: __2__

Each box may contain more than 1 bag.
Count total amount of boxes you need a month. Only order the amount of boxes you have used. Cross out boxes if you use anything less than 60 boxes a month. Grid contains up to 60 boxes a month.

PD Dialysis Supplies Inventory

Count Start Date: __7/19/2022__ Fact #: __123456789__

Quantity in Box														
X	X	X	X	X	X	X	X	X	X	X	X	X	X	X

Item: __cassette__

Qty: __30__

Used: __15__

Left: __15__

Supplies inventory grid goes by quantity per box. Depending on items boxes may contain different amounts.

PD Dialysis Solution Inventory

Count Start Date: _____ **Fact #:** _____

Boxes

Solution Color:

_____

Strength:_____

Liters:_____

Count Start Date: _____ **Fact #:** _____

Boxes

Solution Color:

_____

Strength:_____

Liters:_____

Count Start Date: _____ **Fact #:** _____

Boxes

Solution Color:

_____

Strength:_____

Liters:_____

Count Start Date: _____ **Fact #:** _____

Boxes

Solution Color:

_____

Strength:_____

Liters:_____

Count Start Date: _____ **Fact #:** _____

Boxes

Solution Color:

_____

Strength:_____

Liters:_____

good Vibes Only

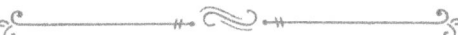

PD Dialysis Solution Inventory

Count Start Date:_____ Fact #:_____

Boxes

Solution Color:

_____

Strength:_____

Liters:_____

Count Start Date:_____ Fact #:_____

Boxes

Solution Color:

_____

Strength:_____

Liters:_____

Count Start Date:_____ Fact #:_____

Boxes

Solution Color:

_____

Strength:_____

Liters:_____

Count Start Date:_____ Fact #:_____

Boxes

Solution Color:

_____

Strength:_____

Liters:_____

Count Start Date:_____ Fact #:_____

Boxes

Solution Color:

_____

Strength:_____

Liters:_____

Don't give up

PD Dialysis Solution Inventory

Count Start Date:_____ Fact #:_____

Boxes

Solution Color:

_____

Strength:_____

Liters:_____

Count Start Date:_____ Fact #:_____

Boxes

Solution Color:

_____

Strength:_____

Liters:_____

Count Start Date:_____ Fact #:_____

Boxes

Solution Color:

_____

Strength:_____

Liters:_____

Count Start Date:_____ Fact #:_____

Boxes

Solution Color:

_____

Strength:_____

Liters:_____

Count Start Date:_____ Fact #:_____

Boxes

Solution Color:

_____

Strength:_____

Liters:_____

Positive thoughts

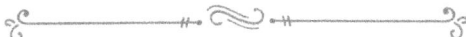

PD Dialysis Solution Inventory

Count Start Date:_____ **Fact #:**_____

Boxes

Solution Color:

_____

Strength:_____

Liters:_____

Count Start Date:_____ **Fact #:**_____

Boxes

Solution Color:

_____

Strength:_____

Liters:_____

Count Start Date:_____ **Fact #:**_____

Boxes

Solution Color:

_____

Strength:_____

Liters:_____

Count Start Date:_____ **Fact #:**_____

Boxes

Solution Color:

_____

Strength:_____

Liters:_____

Count Start Date:_____ **Fact #:**_____

Boxes

Solution Color:

_____

Strength:_____

Liters:_____

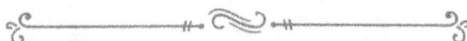

you got this

PD Dialysis Solution Inventory

Count Start Date:_____   Fact #:_____

Boxes

Solution Color:

_____

Strength:_____

Liters:_____

Count Start Date:_____   Fact #:_____

Boxes

Solution Color:

_____

Strength:_____

Liters:_____

Count Start Date:_____   Fact #:_____

Boxes

Solution Color:

_____

Strength:_____

Liters:_____

Count Start Date:_____   Fact #:_____

Boxes

Solution Color:

_____

Strength:_____

Liters:_____

Count Start Date:_____   Fact #:_____

Boxes

Solution Color:

_____

Strength:_____

Liters:_____

I believe in you

PD Dialysis Solution Inventory

Count Start Date:_____ Fact #:_____

Boxes

Solution Color:

_____

Strength:_____

Liters:_____

Count Start Date:_____ Fact #:_____

Boxes

Solution Color:

_____

Strength:_____

Liters:_____

Count Start Date:_____ Fact #:_____

Boxes

Solution Color:

_____

Strength:_____

Liters:_____

Count Start Date:_____ Fact #:_____

Boxes

Solution Color:

_____

Strength:_____

Liters:_____

Count Start Date:_____ Fact #:_____

Boxes

Solution Color:

_____

Strength:_____

Liters:_____

have a good day

PD Dialysis Solution Inventory

Count Start Date:_____ Fact #:_____

Boxes

Solution Color:

_____

Strength:_____

Liters:_____

Count Start Date:_____ Fact #:_____

Boxes

Solution Color:

_____

Strength:_____

Liters:_____

Count Start Date:_____ Fact #:_____

Boxes

Solution Color:

_____

Strength:_____

Liters:_____

Count Start Date:_____ Fact #:_____

Boxes

Solution Color:

_____

Strength:_____

Liters:_____

Count Start Date:_____ Fact #:_____

Boxes

Solution Color:

_____

Strength:_____

Liters:_____

virtual hug

PD Dialysis Solution Inventory

Count Start Date: _____   **Fact #:** _____

Boxes

Solution Color:

_____

Strength: _____

Liters: _____

Count Start Date: _____   **Fact #:** _____

Boxes

Solution Color:

_____

Strength: _____

Liters: _____

Count Start Date: _____   **Fact #:** _____

Boxes

Solution Color:

_____

Strength: _____

Liters: _____

Count Start Date: _____   **Fact #:** _____

Boxes

Solution Color:

_____

Strength: _____

Liters: _____

Count Start Date: _____   **Fact #:** _____

Boxes

Solution Color:

_____

Strength: _____

Liters: _____

it's gonna be ok

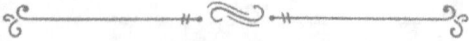

PD Dialysis Solution Inventory

Count Start Date:_____ Fact #:_____

Boxes

Solution Color:

_____

Strength:_____

Liters:_____

Count Start Date:_____ Fact #:_____

Boxes

Solution Color:

_____

Strength:_____

Liters:_____

Count Start Date:_____ Fact #:_____

Boxes

Solution Color:

_____

Strength:_____

Liters:_____

Count Start Date:_____ Fact #:_____

Boxes

Solution Color:

_____

Strength:_____

Liters:_____

Count Start Date:_____ Fact #:_____

Boxes

Solution Color:

_____

Strength:_____

Liters:_____

you are capable of anything

PD Dialysis Solution Inventory

Count Start Date:_____ Fact #:_____

Boxes

Solution Color:

_____

Strength:_____

Liters:_____

Count Start Date:_____ Fact #:_____

Boxes

Solution Color:

_____

Strength:_____

Liters:_____

Count Start Date:_____ Fact #:_____

Boxes

Solution Color:

_____

Strength:_____

Liters:_____

Count Start Date:_____ Fact #:_____

Boxes

Solution Color:

_____

Strength:_____

Liters:_____

Count Start Date:_____ Fact #:_____

Boxes

Solution Color:

_____

Strength:_____

Liters:_____

keep fighting

PD Dialysis Solution Inventory

Count Start Date:_____ Fact #:_____

Boxes

Solution Color:

_____

Strength:_____

Liters:_____

Count Start Date:_____ Fact #:_____

Boxes

Solution Color:

_____

Strength:_____

Liters:_____

Count Start Date:_____ Fact #:_____

Boxes

Solution Color:

_____

Strength:_____

Liters:_____

Count Start Date:_____ Fact #:_____

Boxes

Solution Color:

_____

Strength:_____

Liters:_____

Count Start Date:_____ Fact #:_____

Boxes

Solution Color:

_____

Strength:_____

Liters:_____

you are your super power

PD Dialysis Solution Inventory

Count Start Date: _____ **Fact #:** _____

Boxes

Solution Color:

_____

Strength: _____

Liters: _____

Count Start Date: _____ **Fact #:** _____

Boxes

Solution Color:

_____

Strength: _____

Liters: _____

Count Start Date: _____ **Fact #:** _____

Boxes

Solution Color:

_____

Strength: _____

Liters: _____

Count Start Date: _____ **Fact #:** _____

Boxes

Solution Color:

_____

Strength: _____

Liters: _____

Count Start Date: _____ **Fact #:** _____

Boxes

Solution Color:

_____

Strength: _____

Liters: _____

you're stronger than you think

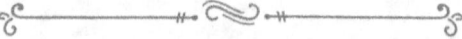

PD Dialysis Solution Inventory

Count Start Date:_____ Fact #:_____

Boxes

Solution Color:
_____
Strength:_____
Liters:_____

Count Start Date:_____ Fact #:_____

Boxes

Solution Color:
_____
Strength:_____
Liters:_____

Count Start Date:_____ Fact #:_____

Boxes

Solution Color:
_____
Strength:_____
Liters:_____

Count Start Date:_____ Fact #:_____

Boxes

Solution Color:
_____
Strength:_____
Liters:_____

Count Start Date:_____ Fact #:_____

Boxes

Solution Color:
_____
Strength:_____
Liters:_____

keep going

PD Dialysis Solution Inventory

Count Start Date:_____ Fact #:_____

Boxes

Solution Color:
_____
Strength:_____
Liters:_____

Count Start Date:_____ Fact #:_____

Boxes

Solution Color:
_____
Strength:_____
Liters:_____

Count Start Date:_____ Fact #:_____

Boxes

Solution Color:
_____
Strength:_____
Liters:_____

Count Start Date:_____ Fact #:_____

Boxes

Solution Color:
_____
Strength:_____
Liters:_____

Count Start Date:_____ Fact #:_____

Boxes

Solution Color:
_____
Strength:_____
Liters:_____

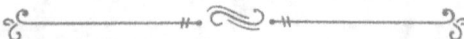

enjoy the little things

PD Dialysis Solution Inventory

Count Start Date:_____ Fact #:_____

Boxes

Solution Color:

_____

Strength:_____

Liters:_____

Count Start Date:_____ Fact #:_____

Boxes

Solution Color:

_____

Strength:_____

Liters:_____

Count Start Date:_____ Fact #:_____

Boxes

Solution Color:

_____

Strength:_____

Liters:_____

Count Start Date:_____ Fact #:_____

Boxes

Solution Color:

_____

Strength:_____

Liters:_____

Count Start Date:_____ Fact #:_____

Boxes

Solution Color:

_____

Strength:_____

Liters:_____

stay healthy

PD Dialysis Solution Inventory

Count Start Date:_____ Fact #:_____

Boxes

Solution Color:
_____
Strength:_____
Liters:_____

Count Start Date:_____ Fact #:_____

Boxes

Solution Color:
_____
Strength:_____
Liters:_____

Count Start Date:_____ Fact #:_____

Boxes

Solution Color:
_____
Strength:_____
Liters:_____

Count Start Date:_____ Fact #:_____

Boxes

Solution Color:
_____
Strength:_____
Liters:_____

Count Start Date:_____ Fact #:_____

Boxes

Solution Color:
_____
Strength:_____
Liters:_____

Good Vibes Only

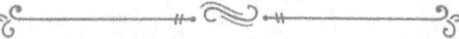

PD Dialysis Solution Inventory

Count Start Date: _____ Fact #: _____

Boxes

Solution Color:

_____

Strength: _____

Liters: _____

Count Start Date: _____ Fact #: _____

Boxes

Solution Color:

_____

Strength: _____

Liters: _____

Count Start Date: _____ Fact #: _____

Boxes

Solution Color:

_____

Strength: _____

Liters: _____

Count Start Date: _____ Fact #: _____

Boxes

Solution Color:

_____

Strength: _____

Liters: _____

Count Start Date: _____ Fact #: _____

Boxes

Solution Color:

_____

Strength: _____

Liters: _____

Don't give up

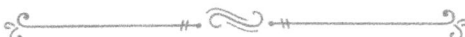

PD Dialysis Solution Inventory

Count Start Date:_____ Fact #:_____

Boxes

Solution Color:

_____

Strength:_____

Liters:_____

Count Start Date:_____ Fact #:_____

Boxes

Solution Color:

_____

Strength:_____

Liters:_____

Count Start Date:_____ Fact #:_____

Boxes

Solution Color:

_____

Strength:_____

Liters:_____

Count Start Date:_____ Fact #:_____

Boxes

Solution Color:

_____

Strength:_____

Liters:_____

Count Start Date:_____ Fact #:_____

Boxes

Solution Color:

_____

Strength:_____

Liters:_____

Positive thoughts

PD Dialysis Solution Inventory

Count Start Date:_____ Fact #:_____

Boxes

Solution Color:

_____

Strength:_____

Liters:_____

Count Start Date:_____ Fact #:_____

Boxes

Solution Color:

_____

Strength:_____

Liters:_____

Count Start Date:_____ Fact #:_____

Boxes

Solution Color:

_____

Strength:_____

Liters:_____

Count Start Date:_____ Fact #:_____

Boxes

Solution Color:

_____

Strength:_____

Liters:_____

Count Start Date:_____ Fact #:_____

Boxes

Solution Color:

_____

Strength:_____

Liters:_____

you got this

PD Dialysis Solution Inventory

Count Start Date:_____ Fact #:_____

Boxes

Solution Color:

_____

Strength:_____

Liters:_____

Count Start Date:_____ Fact #:_____

Boxes

Solution Color:

_____

Strength:_____

Liters:_____

Count Start Date:_____ Fact #:_____

Boxes

Solution Color:

_____

Strength:_____

Liters:_____

Count Start Date:_____ Fact #:_____

Boxes

Solution Color:

_____

Strength:_____

Liters:_____

Count Start Date:_____ Fact #:_____

Boxes

Solution Color:

_____

Strength:_____

Liters:_____

I believe in you

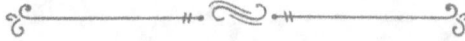

PD Dialysis Solution Inventory

Count Start Date:_____ Fact #:_____

Boxes

Solution Color:

_____

Strength:_____

Liters:_____

Count Start Date:_____ Fact #:_____

Boxes

Solution Color:

_____

Strength:_____

Liters:_____

Count Start Date:_____ Fact #:_____

Boxes

Solution Color:

_____

Strength:_____

Liters:_____

Count Start Date:_____ Fact #:_____

Boxes

Solution Color:

_____

Strength:_____

Liters:_____

Count Start Date:_____ Fact #:_____

Boxes

Solution Color:

_____

Strength:_____

Liters:_____

have a good day

PD Dialysis Solution Inventory

Count Start Date:_____ Fact #:_____

Boxes

Solution Color:

_____

Strength:_____

Liters:_____

Count Start Date:_____ Fact #:_____

Boxes

Solution Color:

_____

Strength:_____

Liters:_____

Count Start Date:_____ Fact #:_____

Boxes

Solution Color:

_____

Strength:_____

Liters:_____

Count Start Date:_____ Fact #:_____

Boxes

Solution Color:

_____

Strength:_____

Liters:_____

Count Start Date:_____ Fact #:_____

Boxes

Solution Color:

_____

Strength:_____

Liters:_____

virtual hug

PD Dialysis Solution Inventory

Count Start Date:_____ Fact #:_____

Boxes

Solution Color:

_____

Strength:_____

Liters:_____

Count Start Date:_____ Fact #:_____

Boxes

Solution Color:

_____

Strength:_____

Liters:_____

Count Start Date:_____ Fact #:_____

Boxes

Solution Color:

_____

Strength:_____

Liters:_____

Count Start Date:_____ Fact #:_____

Boxes

Solution Color:

_____

Strength:_____

Liters:_____

Count Start Date:_____ Fact #:_____

Boxes

Solution Color:

_____

Strength:_____

Liters:_____

it's gonna be ok

PD Dialysis Solution Inventory

Count Start Date:_____ Fact #:_____

Boxes

Solution Color:

_____

Strength:_____

Liters:_____

Count Start Date:_____ Fact #:_____

Boxes

Solution Color:

_____

Strength:_____

Liters:_____

Count Start Date:_____ Fact #:_____

Boxes

Solution Color:

_____

Strength:_____

Liters:_____

Count Start Date:_____ Fact #:_____

Boxes

Solution Color:

_____

Strength:_____

Liters:_____

Count Start Date:_____ Fact #:_____

Boxes

Solution Color:

_____

Strength:_____

Liters:_____

you are capable of anything

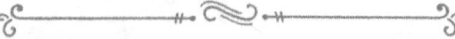

PD Dialysis Solution Inventory

Count Start Date:_____ Fact #:_____

Boxes

Solution Color:

_____

Strength:_____

Liters:_____

Count Start Date:_____ Fact #:_____

Boxes

Solution Color:

_____

Strength:_____

Liters:_____

Count Start Date:_____ Fact #:_____

Boxes

Solution Color:

_____

Strength:_____

Liters:_____

Count Start Date:_____ Fact #:_____

Boxes

Solution Color:

_____

Strength:_____

Liters:_____

Count Start Date:_____ Fact #:_____

Boxes

Solution Color:

_____

Strength:_____

Liters:_____

keep fighting

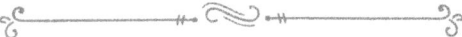

PD Dialysis Solution Inventory

Count Start Date:_____ Fact #:_____

Boxes

Solution Color:

_____

Strength:_____

Liters:_____

Count Start Date:_____ Fact #:_____

Boxes

Solution Color:

_____

Strength:_____

Liters:_____

Count Start Date:_____ Fact #:_____

Boxes

Solution Color:

_____

Strength:_____

Liters:_____

Count Start Date:_____ Fact #:_____

Boxes

Solution Color:

_____

Strength:_____

Liters:_____

Count Start Date:_____ Fact #:_____

Boxes

Solution Color:

_____

Strength:_____

Liters:_____

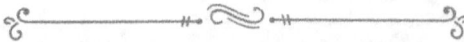

you are your super power

PD Dialysis Solution Inventory

Count Start Date:_____ Fact #:_____

Boxes

Solution Color:
_____
Strength:_____
Liters:_____

Count Start Date:_____ Fact #:_____

Boxes

Solution Color:
_____
Strength:_____
Liters:_____

Count Start Date:_____ Fact #:_____

Boxes

Solution Color:
_____
Strength:_____
Liters:_____

Count Start Date:_____ Fact #:_____

Boxes

Solution Color:
_____
Strength:_____
Liters:_____

Count Start Date:_____ Fact #:_____

Boxes

Solution Color:
_____
Strength:_____
Liters:_____

you're stronger than you think

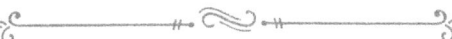

PD Dialysis Solution Inventory

Count Start Date:_____ Fact #:_____

Boxes

Solution Color:

_____

Strength:_____

Liters:_____

Count Start Date:_____ Fact #:_____

Boxes

Solution Color:

_____

Strength:_____

Liters:_____

Count Start Date:_____ Fact #:_____

Boxes

Solution Color:

_____

Strength:_____

Liters:_____

Count Start Date:_____ Fact #:_____

Boxes

Solution Color:

_____

Strength:_____

Liters:_____

Count Start Date:_____ Fact #:_____

Boxes

Solution Color:

_____

Strength:_____

Liters:_____

keep going

PD Dialysis Solution Inventory

Count Start Date:_____ Fact #:_____

Boxes

Solution Color:

_____

Strength:_____

Liters:_____

Count Start Date:_____ Fact #:_____

Boxes

Solution Color:

_____

Strength:_____

Liters:_____

Count Start Date:_____ Fact #:_____

Boxes

Solution Color:

_____

Strength:_____

Liters:_____

Count Start Date:_____ Fact #:_____

Boxes

Solution Color:

_____

Strength:_____

Liters:_____

Count Start Date:_____ Fact #:_____

Boxes

Solution Color:

_____

Strength:_____

Liters:_____

enjoy the little things

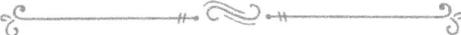

PD Dialysis Solution Inventory

Count Start Date:_____ Fact #:_____

Boxes

Solution Color:
_____

Strength:_____

Liters:_____

Count Start Date:_____ Fact #:_____

Boxes

Solution Color:
_____

Strength:_____

Liters:_____

Count Start Date:_____ Fact #:_____

Boxes

Solution Color:
_____

Strength:_____

Liters:_____

Count Start Date:_____ Fact #:_____

Boxes

Solution Color:
_____

Strength:_____

Liters:_____

Count Start Date:_____ Fact #:_____

Boxes

Solution Color:
_____

Strength:_____

Liters:_____

you're stronger than you think

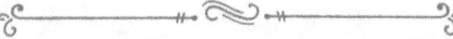

PD Dialysis Solution Inventory

Count Start Date:_____ Fact #:_____

Boxes

Solution Color:
_____
Strength:_____
Liters:_____

Count Start Date:_____ Fact #:_____

Boxes

Solution Color:
_____
Strength:_____
Liters:_____

Count Start Date:_____ Fact #:_____

Boxes

Solution Color:
_____
Strength:_____
Liters:_____

Count Start Date:_____ Fact #:_____

Boxes

Solution Color:
_____
Strength:_____
Liters:_____

Count Start Date:_____ Fact #:_____

Boxes

Solution Color:
_____
Strength:_____
Liters:_____

Good Vibes Only

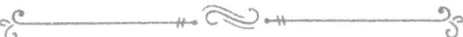

PD Dialysis Solution Inventory

Count Start Date:_____ **Fact #:**_____

Boxes

Solution Color:

_____

Strength:_____

Liters:_____

Count Start Date:_____ **Fact #:**_____

Boxes

Solution Color:

_____

Strength:_____

Liters:_____

Count Start Date:_____ **Fact #:**_____

Boxes

Solution Color:

_____

Strength:_____

Liters:_____

Count Start Date:_____ **Fact #:**_____

Boxes

Solution Color:

_____

Strength:_____

Liters:_____

Count Start Date:_____ **Fact #:**_____

Boxes

Solution Color:

_____

Strength:_____

Liters:_____

Don't give up

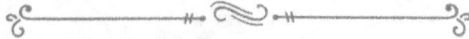

PD Dialysis Solution Inventory

Count Start Date:_____ Fact #:_____

Boxes

Solution Color:

_____

Strength:_____

Liters:_____

Count Start Date:_____ Fact #:_____

Boxes

Solution Color:

_____

Strength:_____

Liters:_____

Count Start Date:_____ Fact #:_____

Boxes

Solution Color:

_____

Strength:_____

Liters:_____

Count Start Date:_____ Fact #:_____

Boxes

Solution Color:

_____

Strength:_____

Liters:_____

Count Start Date:_____ Fact #:_____

Boxes

Solution Color:

_____

Strength:_____

Liters:_____

Positive thoughts

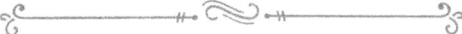

PD Dialysis Solution Inventory

Count Start Date:_____ Fact #:_____

Boxes

Solution Color:

_____

Strength:_____

Liters:_____

Count Start Date:_____ Fact #:_____

Boxes

Solution Color:

_____

Strength:_____

Liters:_____

Count Start Date:_____ Fact #:_____

Boxes

Solution Color:

_____

Strength:_____

Liters:_____

Count Start Date:_____ Fact #:_____

Boxes

Solution Color:

_____

Strength:_____

Liters:_____

Count Start Date:_____ Fact #:_____

Boxes

Solution Color:

_____

Strength:_____

Liters:_____

you got this

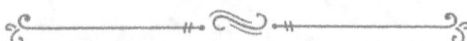

PD Dialysis Solution Inventory

Count Start Date:_____ Fact #:_____

Boxes

Solution Color:

_____

Strength:_____

Liters:_____

Count Start Date:_____ Fact #:_____

Boxes

Solution Color:

_____

Strength:_____

Liters:_____

Count Start Date:_____ Fact #:_____

Boxes

Solution Color:

_____

Strength:_____

Liters:_____

Count Start Date:_____ Fact #:_____

Boxes

Solution Color:

_____

Strength:_____

Liters:_____

Count Start Date:_____ Fact #:_____

Boxes

Solution Color:

_____

Strength:_____

Liters:_____

I believe in you

PD Dialysis Solution Inventory

Count Start Date:_____ Fact #:_____

Boxes

Solution Color:

_____

Strength:_____

Liters:_____

Count Start Date:_____ Fact #:_____

Boxes

Solution Color:

_____

Strength:_____

Liters:_____

Count Start Date:_____ Fact #:_____

Boxes

Solution Color:

_____

Strength:_____

Liters:_____

Count Start Date:_____ Fact #:_____

Boxes

Solution Color:

_____

Strength:_____

Liters:_____

Count Start Date:_____ Fact #:_____

Boxes

Solution Color:

_____

Strength:_____

Liters:_____

have a good day

PD Dialysis Solution Inventory

Count Start Date: _____ Fact #: _____

Boxes

Solution Color: _____

Strength: _____

Liters: _____

Count Start Date: _____ Fact #: _____

Boxes

Solution Color: _____

Strength: _____

Liters: _____

Count Start Date: _____ Fact #: _____

Boxes

Solution Color: _____

Strength: _____

Liters: _____

Count Start Date: _____ Fact #: _____

Boxes

Solution Color: _____

Strength: _____

Liters: _____

Count Start Date: _____ Fact #: _____

Boxes

Solution Color: _____

Strength: _____

Liters: _____

virtual hug

PD Dialysis Solution Inventory

Count Start Date:_____ Fact #:_____

Boxes

Solution Color:

_____

Strength:_____

Liters:_____

Count Start Date:_____ Fact #:_____

Boxes

Solution Color:

_____

Strength:_____

Liters:_____

Count Start Date:_____ Fact #:_____

Boxes

Solution Color:

_____

Strength:_____

Liters:_____

Count Start Date:_____ Fact #:_____

Boxes

Solution Color:

_____

Strength:_____

Liters:_____

Count Start Date:_____ Fact #:_____

Boxes

Solution Color:

_____

Strength:_____

Liters:_____

it's gonna be ok

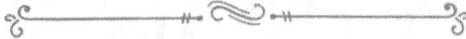

PD Dialysis Solution Inventory

Count Start Date:_____ Fact #:_____

Boxes

Solution Color:
_____

Strength:_____

Liters:_____

Count Start Date:_____ Fact #:_____

Boxes

Solution Color:
_____

Strength:_____

Liters:_____

Count Start Date:_____ Fact #:_____

Boxes

Solution Color:
_____

Strength:_____

Liters:_____

Count Start Date:_____ Fact #:_____

Boxes

Solution Color:
_____

Strength:_____

Liters:_____

Count Start Date:_____ Fact #:_____

Boxes

Solution Color:
_____

Strength:_____

Liters:_____

you are capable of anything

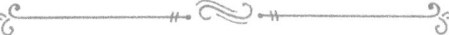

PD Dialysis Solution Inventory

Count Start Date:_____ Fact #:_____

Boxes

Solution Color:
_____

Strength:_____

Liters:_____

Count Start Date:_____ Fact #:_____

Boxes

Solution Color:
_____

Strength:_____

Liters:_____

Count Start Date:_____ Fact #:_____

Boxes

Solution Color:
_____

Strength:_____

Liters:_____

Count Start Date:_____ Fact #:_____

Boxes

Solution Color:
_____

Strength:_____

Liters:_____

Count Start Date:_____ Fact #:_____

Boxes

Solution Color:
_____

Strength:_____

Liters:_____

keep fighting

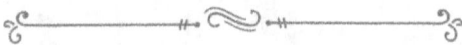

PD Dialysis Supplies Inventory

Count Start Date:_____ Fact #:_____

Quantity in Box

Item:_____
Qty:_____
Used:_____
Left:_____

Count Start Date:_____ Fact #:_____

Quantity in Box

Item:_____
Qty:_____
Used:_____
Left:_____

Count Start Date:_____ Fact #:_____

Quantity in Box

Item:_____
Qty:_____
Used:_____
Left:_____

Count Start Date:_____ Fact #:_____

Quantity in Box

Item:_____
Qty:_____
Used:_____
Left:_____

Count Start Date:_____ Fact #:_____

Quantity in Box

Item:_____
Qty:_____
Used:_____
Left:_____

Count Start Date:_____ Fact #:_____

Quantity in Box

Item:_____
Qty:_____
Used:_____
Left:_____

PD Dialysis Supplies Inventory

Count Start Date:_____ Fact #:_____

Quantity in Box

Item:_____
Qty:_____
Used:_____
Left:_____

Count Start Date:_____ Fact #:_____

Quantity in Box

Item:_____
Qty:_____
Used:_____
Left:_____

Count Start Date:_____ Fact #:_____

Quantity in Box

Item:_____
Qty:_____
Used:_____
Left:_____

Count Start Date:_____ Fact #:_____

Quantity in Box

Item:_____
Qty:_____
Used:_____
Left:_____

Count Start Date:_____ Fact #:_____

Quantity in Box

Item:_____
Qty:_____
Used:_____
Left:_____

Count Start Date:_____ Fact #:_____

Quantity in Box

Item:_____
Qty:_____
Used:_____
Left:_____

PD Dialysis Supplies Inventory

Count Start Date:_____ Fact #:_____

Quantity in Box

Item:_____
Qty:_____
Used:_____
Left:_____

Count Start Date:_____ Fact #:_____

Quantity in Box

Item:_____
Qty:_____
Used:_____
Left:_____

Count Start Date:_____ Fact #:_____

Quantity in Box

Item:_____
Qty:_____
Used:_____
Left:_____

Count Start Date:_____ Fact #:_____

Quantity in Box

Item:_____
Qty:_____
Used:_____
Left:_____

Count Start Date:_____ Fact #:_____

Quantity in Box

Item:_____
Qty:_____
Used:_____
Left:_____

Count Start Date:_____ Fact #:_____

Quantity in Box

Item:_____
Qty:_____
Used:_____
Left:_____

PD Dialysis Supplies Inventory

Count Start Date:_____ Fact #:_____

Quantity in Box

Item:_____
Qty:_____
Used:_____
Left:_____

Count Start Date:_____ Fact #:_____

Quantity in Box

Item:_____
Qty:_____
Used:_____
Left:_____

Count Start Date:_____ Fact #:_____

Quantity in Box

Item:_____
Qty:_____
Used:_____
Left:_____

Count Start Date:_____ Fact #:_____

Quantity in Box

Item:_____
Qty:_____
Used:_____
Left:_____

Count Start Date:_____ Fact #:_____

Quantity in Box

Item:_____
Qty:_____
Used:_____
Left:_____

Count Start Date:_____ Fact #:_____

Quantity in Box

Item:_____
Qty:_____
Used:_____
Left:_____

PD Dialysis Supplies Inventory

Count Start Date:_____ Fact #:_____

Quantity in Box

Item:_____
Qty:_____
Used:_____
Left:_____

Count Start Date:_____ Fact #:_____

Quantity in Box

Item:_____
Qty:_____
Used:_____
Left:_____

Count Start Date:_____ Fact #:_____

Quantity in Box

Item:_____
Qty:_____
Used:_____
Left:_____

Count Start Date:_____ Fact #:_____

Quantity in Box

Item:_____
Qty:_____
Used:_____
Left:_____

Count Start Date:_____ Fact #:_____

Quantity in Box

Item:_____
Qty:_____
Used:_____
Left:_____

Count Start Date:_____ Fact #:_____

Quantity in Box

Item:_____
Qty:_____
Used:_____
Left:_____

PD Dialysis Supplies Inventory

Count Start Date:_____ Fact #:_____

Quantity in Box

Item:_____
Qty:_____
Used:_____
Left:_____

Count Start Date:_____ Fact #:_____

Quantity in Box

Item:_____
Qty:_____
Used:_____
Left:_____

Count Start Date:_____ Fact #:_____

Quantity in Box

Item:_____
Qty:_____
Used:_____
Left:_____

Count Start Date:_____ Fact #:_____

Quantity in Box

Item:_____
Qty:_____
Used:_____
Left:_____

Count Start Date:_____ Fact #:_____

Quantity in Box

Item:_____
Qty:_____
Used:_____
Left:_____

Count Start Date:_____ Fact #:_____

Quantity in Box

Item:_____
Qty:_____
Used:_____
Left:_____

PD Dialysis Supplies Inventory

Count Start Date:_____ Fact #:_____

Quantity in Box

Item:_____
Qty:_____
Used:_____
Left:_____

Count Start Date:_____ Fact #:_____

Quantity in Box

Item:_____
Qty:_____
Used:_____
Left:_____

Count Start Date:_____ Fact #:_____

Quantity in Box

Item:_____
Qty:_____
Used:_____
Left:_____

Count Start Date:_____ Fact #:_____

Quantity in Box

Item:_____
Qty:_____
Used:_____
Left:_____

Count Start Date:_____ Fact #:_____

Quantity in Box

Item:_____
Qty:_____
Used:_____
Left:_____

Count Start Date:_____ Fact #:_____

Quantity in Box

Item:_____
Qty:_____
Used:_____
Left:_____

PD Dialysis Supplies Inventory

Count Start Date:_____ Fact #:_____

Quantity in Box

Item:_____
Qty:_____
Used:_____
Left:_____

Count Start Date:_____ Fact #:_____

Quantity in Box

Item:_____
Qty:_____
Used:_____
Left:_____

Count Start Date:_____ Fact #:_____

Quantity in Box

Item:_____
Qty:_____
Used:_____
Left:_____

Count Start Date:_____ Fact #:_____

Quantity in Box

Item:_____
Qty:_____
Used:_____
Left:_____

Count Start Date:_____ Fact #:_____

Quantity in Box

Item:_____
Qty:_____
Used:_____
Left:_____

Count Start Date:_____ Fact #:_____

Quantity in Box

Item:_____
Qty:_____
Used:_____
Left:_____

PD Dialysis Supplies Inventory

Count Start Date:_____ Fact #:_____

Quantity in Box

Item:_____
Qty:_____
Used:_____
Left:_____

Count Start Date:_____ Fact #:_____

Quantity in Box

Item:_____
Qty:_____
Used:_____
Left:_____

Count Start Date:_____ Fact #:_____

Quantity in Box

Item:_____
Qty:_____
Used:_____
Left:_____

Count Start Date:_____ Fact #:_____

Quantity in Box

Item:_____
Qty:_____
Used:_____
Left:_____

Count Start Date:_____ Fact #:_____

Quantity in Box

Item:_____
Qty:_____
Used:_____
Left:_____

Count Start Date:_____ Fact #:_____

Quantity in Box

Item:_____
Qty:_____
Used:_____
Left:_____

PD Dialysis Supplies Inventory

Count Start Date:_____ Fact #:_____

Quantity in Box

Item:_____
Qty:_____
Used:_____
Left:_____

Count Start Date:_____ Fact #:_____

Quantity in Box

Item:_____
Qty:_____
Used:_____
Left:_____

Count Start Date:_____ Fact #:_____

Quantity in Box

Item:_____
Qty:_____
Used:_____
Left:_____

Count Start Date:_____ Fact #:_____

Quantity in Box

Item:_____
Qty:_____
Used:_____
Left:_____

Count Start Date:_____ Fact #:_____

Quantity in Box

Item:_____
Qty:_____
Used:_____
Left:_____

Count Start Date:_____ Fact #:_____

Quantity in Box

Item:_____
Qty:_____
Used:_____
Left:_____

PD Dialysis Supplies Inventory

Count Start Date:_____ Fact #:_____

Quantity in Box

Item:_____
Qty:_____
Used:_____
Left:_____

Count Start Date:_____ Fact #:_____

Quantity in Box

Item:_____
Qty:_____
Used:_____
Left:_____

Count Start Date:_____ Fact #:_____

Quantity in Box

Item:_____
Qty:_____
Used:_____
Left:_____

Count Start Date:_____ Fact #:_____

Quantity in Box

Item:_____
Qty:_____
Used:_____
Left:_____

Count Start Date:_____ Fact #:_____

Quantity in Box

Item:_____
Qty:_____
Used:_____
Left:_____

Count Start Date:_____ Fact #:_____

Quantity in Box

Item:_____
Qty:_____
Used:_____
Left:_____

PD Dialysis Supplies Inventory

Count Start Date:_____ Fact #:_____

Quantity in Box

Item:_____
Qty:_____
Used:_____
Left:_____

Count Start Date:_____ Fact #:_____

Quantity in Box

Item:_____
Qty:_____
Used:_____
Left:_____

Count Start Date:_____ Fact #:_____

Quantity in Box

Item:_____
Qty:_____
Used:_____
Left:_____

Count Start Date:_____ Fact #:_____

Quantity in Box

Item:_____
Qty:_____
Used:_____
Left:_____

Count Start Date:_____ Fact #:_____

Quantity in Box

Item:_____
Qty:_____
Used:_____
Left:_____

Count Start Date:_____ Fact #:_____

Quantity in Box

Item:_____
Qty:_____
Used:_____
Left:_____

PD Dialysis Supplies Inventory

Count Start Date:_____ Fact #:_____

Quantity in Box

Item:_____
Qty:_____
Used:_____
Left:_____

Count Start Date:_____ Fact #:_____

Quantity in Box

Item:_____
Qty:_____
Used:_____
Left:_____

Count Start Date:_____ Fact #:_____

Quantity in Box

Item:_____
Qty:_____
Used:_____
Left:_____

Count Start Date:_____ Fact #:_____

Quantity in Box

Item:_____
Qty:_____
Used:_____
Left:_____

Count Start Date:_____ Fact #:_____

Quantity in Box

Item:_____
Qty:_____
Used:_____
Left:_____

Count Start Date:_____ Fact #:_____

Quantity in Box

Item:_____
Qty:_____
Used:_____
Left:_____

PD Dialysis Supplies Inventory

Count Start Date: _____ **Fact #:** _____

Quantity in Box

Item: _____
Qty: _____
Used: _____
Left: _____

Count Start Date: _____ **Fact #:** _____

Quantity in Box

Item: _____
Qty: _____
Used: _____
Left: _____

Count Start Date: _____ **Fact #:** _____

Quantity in Box

Item: _____
Qty: _____
Used: _____
Left: _____

Count Start Date: _____ **Fact #:** _____

Quantity in Box

Item: _____
Qty: _____
Used: _____
Left: _____

Count Start Date: _____ **Fact #:** _____

Quantity in Box

Item: _____
Qty: _____
Used: _____
Left: _____

Count Start Date: _____ **Fact #:** _____

Quantity in Box

Item: _____
Qty: _____
Used: _____
Left: _____

PD Dialysis Supplies Inventory

Count Start Date:_____ Fact #:_____

Quantity in Box

Item:_____
Qty:_____
Used:_____
Left:_____

Count Start Date:_____ Fact #:_____

Quantity in Box

Item:_____
Qty:_____
Used:_____
Left:_____

Count Start Date:_____ Fact #:_____

Quantity in Box

Item:_____
Qty:_____
Used:_____
Left:_____

Count Start Date:_____ Fact #:_____

Quantity in Box

Item:_____
Qty:_____
Used:_____
Left:_____

Count Start Date:_____ Fact #:_____

Quantity in Box

Item:_____
Qty:_____
Used:_____
Left:_____

Count Start Date:_____ Fact #:_____

Quantity in Box

Item:_____
Qty:_____
Used:_____
Left:_____

PD Dialysis Supplies Inventory

Count Start Date:_____ Fact #:_____

Quantity in Box

Item:_____
Qty:_____
Used:_____
Left:_____

Count Start Date:_____ Fact #:_____

Quantity in Box

Item:_____
Qty:_____
Used:_____
Left:_____

Count Start Date:_____ Fact #:_____

Quantity in Box

Item:_____
Qty:_____
Used:_____
Left:_____

Count Start Date:_____ Fact #:_____

Quantity in Box

Item:_____
Qty:_____
Used:_____
Left:_____

Count Start Date:_____ Fact #:_____

Quantity in Box

Item:_____
Qty:_____
Used:_____
Left:_____

Count Start Date:_____ Fact #:_____

Quantity in Box

Item:_____
Qty:_____
Used:_____
Left:_____

PD Dialysis Supplies Inventory

Count Start Date:_____   Fact #:_____

Quantity in Box

Item:_____
Qty:_____
Used:_____
Left:_____

Count Start Date:_____   Fact #:_____

Quantity in Box

Item:_____
Qty:_____
Used:_____
Left:_____

Count Start Date:_____   Fact #:_____

Quantity in Box

Item:_____
Qty:_____
Used:_____
Left:_____

Count Start Date:_____   Fact #:_____

Quantity in Box

Item:_____
Qty:_____
Used:_____
Left:_____

Count Start Date:_____   Fact #:_____

Quantity in Box

Item:_____
Qty:_____
Used:_____
Left:_____

Count Start Date:_____   Fact #:_____

Quantity in Box

Item:_____
Qty:_____
Used:_____
Left:_____

PD Dialysis Supplies Inventory

Count Start Date:_____ Fact #:_____

Quantity in Box

Item:_____
Qty:_____
Used:_____
Left:_____

Count Start Date:_____ Fact #:_____

Quantity in Box

Item:_____
Qty:_____
Used:_____
Left:_____

Count Start Date:_____ Fact #:_____

Quantity in Box

Item:_____
Qty:_____
Used:_____
Left:_____

Count Start Date:_____ Fact #:_____

Quantity in Box

Item:_____
Qty:_____
Used:_____
Left:_____

Count Start Date:_____ Fact #:_____

Quantity in Box

Item:_____
Qty:_____
Used:_____
Left:_____

Count Start Date:_____ Fact #:_____

Quantity in Box

Item:_____
Qty:_____
Used:_____
Left:_____

PD Dialysis Supplies Inventory

Count Start Date:_____ **Fact #:**_____

Quantity in Box

Item:_____
Qty:_____
Used:_____
Left:_____

Count Start Date:_____ **Fact #:**_____

Quantity in Box

Item:_____
Qty:_____
Used:_____
Left:_____

Count Start Date:_____ **Fact #:**_____

Quantity in Box

Item:_____
Qty:_____
Used:_____
Left:_____

Count Start Date:_____ **Fact #:**_____

Quantity in Box

Item:_____
Qty:_____
Used:_____
Left:_____

Count Start Date:_____ **Fact #:**_____

Quantity in Box

Item:_____
Qty:_____
Used:_____
Left:_____

Count Start Date:_____ **Fact #:**_____

Quantity in Box

Item:_____
Qty:_____
Used:_____
Left:_____

PD Dialysis Supplies Inventory

Count Start Date: _____ **Fact #:** _____

Quantity in Box

Item:_____
Qty:_____
Used:_____
Left:_____

Count Start Date: _____ **Fact #:** _____

Quantity in Box

Item:_____
Qty:_____
Used:_____
Left:_____

Count Start Date: _____ **Fact #:** _____

Quantity in Box

Item:_____
Qty:_____
Used:_____
Left:_____

Count Start Date: _____ **Fact #:** _____

Quantity in Box

Item:_____
Qty:_____
Used:_____
Left:_____

Count Start Date: _____ **Fact #:** _____

Quantity in Box

Item:_____
Qty:_____
Used:_____
Left:_____

Count Start Date: _____ **Fact #:** _____

Quantity in Box

Item:_____
Qty:_____
Used:_____
Left:_____

PD Dialysis Supplies Inventory

Count Start Date:_____ Fact #:_____

Quantity in Box

Item:_____
Qty:_____
Used:_____
Left:_____

Count Start Date:_____ Fact #:_____

Quantity in Box

Item:_____
Qty:_____
Used:_____
Left:_____

Count Start Date:_____ Fact #:_____

Quantity in Box

Item:_____
Qty:_____
Used:_____
Left:_____

Count Start Date:_____ Fact #:_____

Quantity in Box

Item:_____
Qty:_____
Used:_____
Left:_____

Count Start Date:_____ Fact #:_____

Quantity in Box

Item:_____
Qty:_____
Used:_____
Left:_____

Count Start Date:_____ Fact #:_____

Quantity in Box

Item:_____
Qty:_____
Used:_____
Left:_____

PD Dialysis Supplies Inventory

Count Start Date:_____   Fact #:_____

Quantity in Box

Item:_____
Qty:_____
Used:_____
Left:_____

Count Start Date:_____   Fact #:_____

Quantity in Box

Item:_____
Qty:_____
Used:_____
Left:_____

Count Start Date:_____   Fact #:_____

Quantity in Box

Item:_____
Qty:_____
Used:_____
Left:_____

Count Start Date:_____   Fact #:_____

Quantity in Box

Item:_____
Qty:_____
Used:_____
Left:_____

Count Start Date:_____   Fact #:_____

Quantity in Box

Item:_____
Qty:_____
Used:_____
Left:_____

Count Start Date:_____   Fact #:_____

Quantity in Box

Item:_____
Qty:_____
Used:_____
Left:_____

PD Dialysis Supplies Inventory

Count Start Date:_____ **Fact #:**_____

Quantity in Box

Item:_____
Qty:_____
Used:_____
Left:_____

Count Start Date:_____ **Fact #:**_____

Quantity in Box

Item:_____
Qty:_____
Used:_____
Left:_____

Count Start Date:_____ **Fact #:**_____

Quantity in Box

Item:_____
Qty:_____
Used:_____
Left:_____

Count Start Date:_____ **Fact #:**_____

Quantity in Box

Item:_____
Qty:_____
Used:_____
Left:_____

Count Start Date:_____ **Fact #:**_____

Quantity in Box

Item:_____
Qty:_____
Used:_____
Left:_____

Count Start Date:_____ **Fact #:**_____

Quantity in Box

Item:_____
Qty:_____
Used:_____
Left:_____

PD Dialysis Supplies Inventory

Count Start Date:_____ Fact #:_____

Quantity in Box

Item:_____
Qty:_____
Used:_____
Left:_____

Count Start Date:_____ Fact #:_____

Quantity in Box

Item:_____
Qty:_____
Used:_____
Left:_____

Count Start Date:_____ Fact #:_____

Quantity in Box

Item:_____
Qty:_____
Used:_____
Left:_____

Count Start Date:_____ Fact #:_____

Quantity in Box

Item:_____
Qty:_____
Used:_____
Left:_____

Count Start Date:_____ Fact #:_____

Quantity in Box

Item:_____
Qty:_____
Used:_____
Left:_____

Count Start Date:_____ Fact #:_____

Quantity in Box

Item:_____
Qty:_____
Used:_____
Left:_____

PD Dialysis Supplies Inventory

Count Start Date:_____ Fact #:_____

Quantity in Box

Item:_____
Qty:_____
Used:_____
Left:_____

Count Start Date:_____ Fact #:_____

Quantity in Box

Item:_____
Qty:_____
Used:_____
Left:_____

Count Start Date:_____ Fact #:_____

Quantity in Box

Item:_____
Qty:_____
Used:_____
Left:_____

Count Start Date:_____ Fact #:_____

Quantity in Box

Item:_____
Qty:_____
Used:_____
Left:_____

Count Start Date:_____ Fact #:_____

Quantity in Box

Item:_____
Qty:_____
Used:_____
Left:_____

Count Start Date:_____ Fact #:_____

Quantity in Box

Item:_____
Qty:_____
Used:_____
Left:_____

PD Dialysis Supplies Inventory

Count Start Date:_____ Fact #:_____

Quantity in Box

Item:_____
Qty:_____
Used:_____
Left:_____

Count Start Date:_____ Fact #:_____

Quantity in Box

Item:_____
Qty:_____
Used:_____
Left:_____

Count Start Date:_____ Fact #:_____

Quantity in Box

Item:_____
Qty:_____
Used:_____
Left:_____

Count Start Date:_____ Fact #:_____

Quantity in Box

Item:_____
Qty:_____
Used:_____
Left:_____

Count Start Date:_____ Fact #:_____

Quantity in Box

Item:_____
Qty:_____
Used:_____
Left:_____

Count Start Date:_____ Fact #:_____

Quantity in Box

Item:_____
Qty:_____
Used:_____
Left:_____

PD Dialysis Supplies Inventory

Count Start Date:_____ Fact #:_____

Quantity in Box

Item:_____
Qty:_____
Used:_____
Left:_____

Count Start Date:_____ Fact #:_____

Quantity in Box

Item:_____
Qty:_____
Used:_____
Left:_____

Count Start Date:_____ Fact #:_____

Quantity in Box

Item:_____
Qty:_____
Used:_____
Left:_____

Count Start Date:_____ Fact #:_____

Quantity in Box

Item:_____
Qty:_____
Used:_____
Left:_____

Count Start Date:_____ Fact #:_____

Quantity in Box

Item:_____
Qty:_____
Used:_____
Left:_____

Count Start Date:_____ Fact #:_____

Quantity in Box

Item:_____
Qty:_____
Used:_____
Left:_____

PD Dialysis Supplies Inventory

Count Start Date:_____ Fact #:_____

Quantity in Box

Item:_____
Qty:_____
Used:_____
Left:_____

Count Start Date:_____ Fact #:_____

Quantity in Box

Item:_____
Qty:_____
Used:_____
Left:_____

Count Start Date:_____ Fact #:_____

Quantity in Box

Item:_____
Qty:_____
Used:_____
Left:_____

Count Start Date:_____ Fact #:_____

Quantity in Box

Item:_____
Qty:_____
Used:_____
Left:_____

Count Start Date:_____ Fact #:_____

Quantity in Box

Item:_____
Qty:_____
Used:_____
Left:_____

Count Start Date:_____ Fact #:_____

Quantity in Box

Item:_____
Qty:_____
Used:_____
Left:_____

PD Dialysis Supplies Inventory

Count Start Date:_____ Fact #:_____

Quantity in Box

Item:_____
Qty:_____
Used:_____
Left:_____

Count Start Date:_____ Fact #:_____

Quantity in Box

Item:_____
Qty:_____
Used:_____
Left:_____

Count Start Date:_____ Fact #:_____

Quantity in Box

Item:_____
Qty:_____
Used:_____
Left:_____

Count Start Date:_____ Fact #:_____

Quantity in Box

Item:_____
Qty:_____
Used:_____
Left:_____

Count Start Date:_____ Fact #:_____

Quantity in Box

Item:_____
Qty:_____
Used:_____
Left:_____

Count Start Date:_____ Fact #:_____

Quantity in Box

Item:_____
Qty:_____
Used:_____
Left:_____

PD Dialysis Supplies Inventory

Count Start Date:_____ Fact #:_____

Quantity in Box

Item:_____
Qty:_____
Used:_____
Left:_____

Count Start Date:_____ Fact #:_____

Quantity in Box

Item:_____
Qty:_____
Used:_____
Left:_____

Count Start Date:_____ Fact #:_____

Quantity in Box

Item:_____
Qty:_____
Used:_____
Left:_____

Count Start Date:_____ Fact #:_____

Quantity in Box

Item:_____
Qty:_____
Used:_____
Left:_____

Count Start Date:_____ Fact #:_____

Quantity in Box

Item:_____
Qty:_____
Used:_____
Left:_____

Count Start Date:_____ Fact #:_____

Quantity in Box

Item:_____
Qty:_____
Used:_____
Left:_____

PD Dialysis Supplies Inventory

Count Start Date:_____ Fact #:_____

Quantity in Box

Item:_____
Qty:_____
Used:_____
Left:_____

Count Start Date:_____ Fact #:_____

Quantity in Box

Item:_____
Qty:_____
Used:_____
Left:_____

Count Start Date:_____ Fact #:_____

Quantity in Box

Item:_____
Qty:_____
Used:_____
Left:_____

Count Start Date:_____ Fact #:_____

Quantity in Box

Item:_____
Qty:_____
Used:_____
Left:_____

Count Start Date:_____ Fact #:_____

Quantity in Box

Item:_____
Qty:_____
Used:_____
Left:_____

Count Start Date:_____ Fact #:_____

Quantity in Box

Item:_____
Qty:_____
Used:_____
Left:_____

PD Dialysis Supplies Inventory

Count Start Date:_____ Fact #:_____

Quantity in Box

Item:_____
Qty:_____
Used:_____
Left:_____

Count Start Date:_____ Fact #:_____

Quantity in Box

Item:_____
Qty:_____
Used:_____
Left:_____

Count Start Date:_____ Fact #:_____

Quantity in Box

Item:_____
Qty:_____
Used:_____
Left:_____

Count Start Date:_____ Fact #:_____

Quantity in Box

Item:_____
Qty:_____
Used:_____
Left:_____

Count Start Date:_____ Fact #:_____

Quantity in Box

Item:_____
Qty:_____
Used:_____
Left:_____

Count Start Date:_____ Fact #:_____

Quantity in Box

Item:_____
Qty:_____
Used:_____
Left:_____

PD Dialysis Supplies Inventory

Count Start Date:_____ Fact #:_____

Quantity in Box

Item:_____
Qty:_____
Used:_____
Left:_____

Count Start Date:_____ Fact #:_____

Quantity in Box

Item:_____
Qty:_____
Used:_____
Left:_____

Count Start Date:_____ Fact #:_____

Quantity in Box

Item:_____
Qty:_____
Used:_____
Left:_____

Count Start Date:_____ Fact #:_____

Quantity in Box

Item:_____
Qty:_____
Used:_____
Left:_____

Count Start Date:_____ Fact #:_____

Quantity in Box

Item:_____
Qty:_____
Used:_____
Left:_____

Count Start Date:_____ Fact #:_____

Quantity in Box

Item:_____
Qty:_____
Used:_____
Left:_____

PD Dialysis Supplies Inventory

Count Start Date:_____ Fact #:_____

Quantity in Box

Item:_____
Qty:_____
Used:_____
Left:_____

Count Start Date:_____ Fact #:_____

Quantity in Box

Item:_____
Qty:_____
Used:_____
Left:_____

Count Start Date:_____ Fact #:_____

Quantity in Box

Item:_____
Qty:_____
Used:_____
Left:_____

Count Start Date:_____ Fact #:_____

Quantity in Box

Item:_____
Qty:_____
Used:_____
Left:_____

Count Start Date:_____ Fact #:_____

Quantity in Box

Item:_____
Qty:_____
Used:_____
Left:_____

Count Start Date:_____ Fact #:_____

Quantity in Box

Item:_____
Qty:_____
Used:_____
Left:_____

PD Dialysis Supplies Inventory

Count Start Date:_____ Fact #:_____

Quantity in Box

Item:_____
Qty:_____
Used:_____
Left:_____

Count Start Date:_____ Fact #:_____

Quantity in Box

Item:_____
Qty:_____
Used:_____
Left:_____

Count Start Date:_____ Fact #:_____

Quantity in Box

Item:_____
Qty:_____
Used:_____
Left:_____

Count Start Date:_____ Fact #:_____

Quantity in Box

Item:_____
Qty:_____
Used:_____
Left:_____

Count Start Date:_____ Fact #:_____

Quantity in Box

Item:_____
Qty:_____
Used:_____
Left:_____

Count Start Date:_____ Fact #:_____

Quantity in Box

Item:_____
Qty:_____
Used:_____
Left:_____

PD Dialysis Supplies Inventory

Count Start Date:_____   Fact #:_____

Quantity in Box

Item:_____
Qty:_____
Used:_____
Left:_____

Count Start Date:_____   Fact #:_____

Quantity in Box

Item:_____
Qty:_____
Used:_____
Left:_____

Count Start Date:_____   Fact #:_____

Quantity in Box

Item:_____
Qty:_____
Used:_____
Left:_____

Count Start Date:_____   Fact #:_____

Quantity in Box

Item:_____
Qty:_____
Used:_____
Left:_____

Count Start Date:_____   Fact #:_____

Quantity in Box

Item:_____
Qty:_____
Used:_____
Left:_____

Count Start Date:_____   Fact #:_____

Quantity in Box

Item:_____
Qty:_____
Used:_____
Left:_____

PD Dialysis Supplies Inventory

Count Start Date:_____ Fact #:_____

Quantity in Box

Item:_____
Qty:_____
Used:_____
Left:_____

Count Start Date:_____ Fact #:_____

Quantity in Box

Item:_____
Qty:_____
Used:_____
Left:_____

Count Start Date:_____ Fact #:_____

Quantity in Box

Item:_____
Qty:_____
Used:_____
Left:_____

Count Start Date:_____ Fact #:_____

Quantity in Box

Item:_____
Qty:_____
Used:_____
Left:_____

Count Start Date:_____ Fact #:_____

Quantity in Box

Item:_____
Qty:_____
Used:_____
Left:_____

Count Start Date:_____ Fact #:_____

Quantity in Box

Item:_____
Qty:_____
Used:_____
Left:_____

PD Dialysis Supplies Inventory

Count Start Date:_____ Fact #:_____

Quantity in Box

Item:_____
Qty:_____
Used:_____
Left:_____

Count Start Date:_____ Fact #:_____

Quantity in Box

Item:_____
Qty:_____
Used:_____
Left:_____

Count Start Date:_____ Fact #:_____

Quantity in Box

Item:_____
Qty:_____
Used:_____
Left:_____

Count Start Date:_____ Fact #:_____

Quantity in Box

Item:_____
Qty:_____
Used:_____
Left:_____

Count Start Date:_____ Fact #:_____

Quantity in Box

Item:_____
Qty:_____
Used:_____
Left:_____

Count Start Date:_____ Fact #:_____

Quantity in Box

Item:_____
Qty:_____
Used:_____
Left:_____

PD Dialysis Supplies Inventory

Count Start Date:_____ Fact #:_____

Quantity in Box

Item:_____
Qty:_____
Used:_____
Left:_____

Count Start Date:_____ Fact #:_____

Quantity in Box

Item:_____
Qty:_____
Used:_____
Left:_____

Count Start Date:_____ Fact #:_____

Quantity in Box

Item:_____
Qty:_____
Used:_____
Left:_____

Count Start Date:_____ Fact #:_____

Quantity in Box

Item:_____
Qty:_____
Used:_____
Left:_____

Count Start Date:_____ Fact #:_____

Quantity in Box

Item:_____
Qty:_____
Used:_____
Left:_____

Count Start Date:_____ Fact #:_____

Quantity in Box

Item:_____
Qty:_____
Used:_____
Left:_____

PD Dialysis Supplies Inventory

Count Start Date:_____ Fact #:_____

Quantity in Box

Item:_____
Qty:_____
Used:_____
Left:_____

Count Start Date:_____ Fact #:_____

Quantity in Box

Item:_____
Qty:_____
Used:_____
Left:_____

Count Start Date:_____ Fact #:_____

Quantity in Box

Item:_____
Qty:_____
Used:_____
Left:_____

Count Start Date:_____ Fact #:_____

Quantity in Box

Item:_____
Qty:_____
Used:_____
Left:_____

Count Start Date:_____ Fact #:_____

Quantity in Box

Item:_____
Qty:_____
Used:_____
Left:_____

Count Start Date:_____ Fact #:_____

Quantity in Box

Item:_____
Qty:_____
Used:_____
Left:_____

PD Dialysis

Notes

Questions

O

O

O

O

O

O

O

Concerns

O

O

O

O

PD Dialysis

Notes

_____
_____
_____
_____
_____
_____
_____
_____
_____

Questions

O _____

O _____

O _____

O _____

O _____

O _____

O _____

Concerns

O _____

O _____

O _____

O _____

PD Dialysis

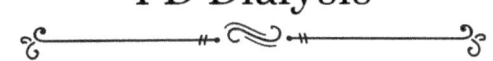

Notes

Questions

o

o

o

o

o

o

o

Concerns

o

o

o

o

PD Dialysis

Notes

Questions
o

o

o

o

o

o

o

Concerns
o

o

o

o

PD Dialysis

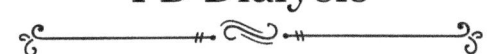

Notes

Questions

O

O

O

O

O

O

O

Concerns

O

O

O

O

PD Dialysis

Notes

Questions

O

O

O

O

O

O

O

Concerns

O

O

O

O

PD Dialysis

Notes

Questions

O

O

O

O

O

O

O

Concerns

O

O

O

O

PD Dialysis

Notes

_____

_____

_____

_____

_____

_____

_____

_____

Questions

o _____

o _____

o _____

o _____

o _____

o _____

o _____

Concerns

o _____

o _____

o _____

o _____

PD Dialysis

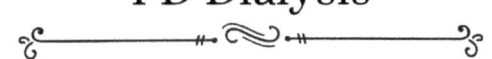

Notes

Questions

o

o

o

o

o

o

o

Concerns

o

o

o

o

PD Dialysis

Notes

_____

_____

_____

_____

_____

_____

_____

_____

Questions

O _____

O _____

O _____

O _____

O _____

O _____

O _____

Concerns

O _____

O _____

O _____

O _____

PD Dialysis

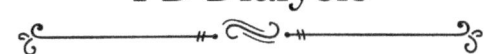

Notes

Questions

o

o

o

o

o

o

o

Concerns

o

o

o

o

PD Dialysis

Notes

Questions

O

O

O

O

O

O

O

Concerns

O

O

O

O

PD Dialysis

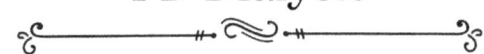

Notes

Questions

O

O

O

O

O

O

O

Concerns

O

O

O

O

PD Dialysis

Notes

_____
_____
_____
_____
_____
_____
_____
_____

Questions

o _____

o _____

o _____

o _____

o _____

o _____

o _____

Concerns

o _____

o _____

o _____

o _____

PD Dialysis

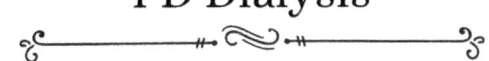

Notes

Questions

o

o

o

o

o

o

o

Concerns

o

o

o

o

PD Dialysis

Notes

_____
_____
_____
_____
_____
_____
_____
_____

Questions

O _____

O _____

O _____

O _____

O _____

O _____

O _____

Concerns

O _____

O _____

O _____

O _____

PD Dialysis

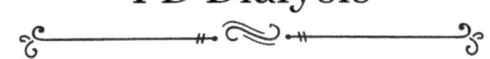

Notes

Questions

o

o

o

o

o

o

o

Concerns

o

o

o

o